# Understanding the Power of Sleeping

## How sleeping better can change your life ?

**Anne Pelland**

# Disclaimer



Disclaimer and Terms of Use: Effort has been made to ensure that the information in this book is accurate and complete, however, the author and the publisher do not warrant the accuracy of the information, text and graphics contained within the book due to the rapidly changing nature of science, research, known and unknown facts, and the internet. The author and publisher assume no liability with respect to losses or damages caused, or alleged to be caused, by any reliance on any information contained herein and disclaim any and all warranties, express or implied, as to the accuracy or reliability of said information.

The publisher and author make no representations or warranties with respect to the accuracy or completeness of the contents of this work and specifically disclaim all warranties. The advice and strategies contained herein may not be suitable for every situation. The Author and the publisher do not hold any responsibility for errors, omissions or contrary interpretation of the subject matter herein. This publication is designed to provide accurate and authoritative information regarding the subject matter covered and is presented solely for motivational and informational purposes only.

Nothing in this book is a substitute for medical advice nor is it intended to diagnose, treat, cure or prevent any illness or health condition. If you have a condition or health problem, consult your personal health care provider. This book is sold with the understanding that neither the author nor the publisher is engaged in rendering professional services.

# Table of Contents

# Sleep - Understand the Basics

Sleep is essential for a person's health and well-being, according to the National Sleep Foundation (NSF). Sleep is as important as food and air. It is a necessary function required to support all human life, growth, development and brain function. Sleep keeps your mind alert and calm. It helps you in optimal daily functioning. If you wake up tired after sleeping for eight hours or longer, more sleep is not what you need. A better quality of sleep is what's needed rather than more sleep. Deep sleep is the most important type of sleep our body needs.

**What is sleep?**

Sleep was long considered just a block of time when you are not awake. But sleep studies done over the past several decades, have discovered that sleep has distinctive stages that cycle throughout the night. Your brain stays active throughout sleep, but different things happen during each stage.

From a medical point of view, sleep can be understood as a state of mind experiencing reduced levels of consciousness involving a temporary inactivity of nearly all voluntary muscles, and a relative suspension of sensory and non-motor activity. In simple terms, sleep is an impermanent physical and mental state of the mind during which most of the external stimuli are blocked from the senses, and the individual stops responding to the environment.

**How much sleep is enough?**

Sleep needs vary from person to person. These needs vary throughout the life-cycle. Most adults need 7-8 hours of sleep each night. Newborns sleep between 16 and 18 hours a day. Children in preschool sleep between 10 and 12 hours a day. However, some individuals are able to function without sleepiness or drowsiness after as little as six hours of sleep. Others can't perform at their peak unless they've slept ten hours.

Some people believe that adults need less sleep as they get older. But there is no evidence to show that older people can get by with less sleep than younger people. Older people are also more easily awakened.

Research suggests that a lot of people can be reassured that six or seven hours sleep is okay. The acid test for enough sleep is whether you are sleepy or alert throughout the day. If you are alert, then your sleep is probably adequate. But sleep is more important than you may think

There are different types of "periods of sleep" depending upon the intensity and manifestation of sleeping criteria. The ability of the person to "awake", or come out from the transitory partial inactive state of the mind depends upon several factors, and these factors vary from person-to-person. Even though it can't be proved on a conclusive basis, medical experts believe the basic purpose of sleep is to create a state of inertness in the human body, during which the body can repair itself and regulate the metabolism to improve its functioning, and the state of inertness helps save the energy which is utilized for the rejuvenation process.

**Repair theory**

As per this theory, during the "awake" period, the body is physically and mentally responding to the various activities associated with our daily activities and this consumes large amounts of energy. The energy utilized is depleted from the energy reserves stored in various parts of the body. The replenishment and body repair activities can occur effectively when the body is undergoing a state of rest - when no extra energy is utilized for any physical processes or activities. The sleep period ensures all the resources in the body are utilized in an optimum manner for the maintenance and upkeep of the various metabolic processes occurring in our body that keep us alive.

**Adaptive theory**

According to this theory, sleep is a naturally evolved phenomenon that humans and animals adapted to for their survival. Sleeping helps in preserving energy and prevents exposure to dangers and predators.

How "sleep" works?

As far as the process of sleeping is concerned, scientists believe that our metabolism has two processes:

• The sleep-wake process

• Circadian biological clock or Circadian rhythm

which regulate our sleep. Both the processes function in tandem, and create the "sleep cycle" because of which we tend to feel sleepy at night, and remain awake during the day. The processes regulate our sleep cycle, which scientists believe is essential for body repair and sustenance. The Circadian biological clock can be understood as a 24-hour condition during which the body rhythm is affected by sunlight. The presence and absence of sunlight control the secretion of certain essential hormones in the body. The melatonin hormone (N-acetyl-5-methoxytryptamine) is secreted in the absence of sunlight, generally at night, and is primarily responsible for regulating the body temperature. The cycle needs to be in accord with the physical state of the individual and the metabolic functioning of the body.

**Circadian rhythm or the "sleep cycle"**

A Circadian rhythm is an approximately 24-hour cycle associated with the biochemical, physiological, and/or behavioral processes. The term "circadian" is derived from the Latin word "circa" which means "around", and "diem" or "dies" which means "day". Therefore, the term literally means "approximately one day". The rhythm is generated by a metabolic activity which functions as an internal body clock, and which is synchronized with the "light-dark" cycles as well as the changes taking place in the subject's environment.

# Sleep and Stages

The sleep process consists of two main stages which keep on repeating in a cycle of 90 to 110 minutes during the entire sleeping activity. The two stages are:

• REM (Rapid Eye Movement)

• Non-REM (Non - Rapid Eye Movement, which is further classified into four substages)

**REM sleep**

The Rapid Eye Movement (REM) stage of sleep is characterized by a rapid movement of the eyes, in addition to a low muscle tone, and/or a partial paralysis of all voluntary muscles. In the case of humans, this type of sleep occupies between 20% to 25% of the total sleep duration which is approximately 90 to 120 minutes. Typically, about four to five cycles occur during normal REM sleep. The duration of the cycle is short at the beginning of the sleep and starts extending towards the end. The exact duration of REM sleep required can't be ascertained since the sleep cycle varies from individual to individual as per the body's metabolic requirements. In the case of newborn babies, the REM stage consists of around 80% of the total sleeping time. REM sleep is also affected by the aging process. During the REM stage, no dominate brain waves are emitted as per polysomnogram findings.

The first REM cycle usually begins approximately 70 to 90 minutes after the sleeping process commences i.e. after falling asleep. During the REM stage, even though the subject is not responsive to any strong external stimuli, the brain remains active, and as per polysomnogram tests, the degree of activity is considerably more as compared to the "awake" stage. The REM stage is also associated with the "dreaming" phenomenon, and when the process occurs, the frequency of REM i.e. the movement of eyes increases significantly. Typically, depending upon the intensity of the dreaming activity, the blood pressure too is affected and can increase marginally or significantly.

**Non-REM sleep**

The Non-REM sleep stage is characterized by an absence of rapid eye movement, a decrease in the metabolic activity, a reduction in the breathing and heart rates, and generally a substantial decrease amounting to almost an absence of dreaming activity. Unlike the REM stage, voluntary muscles do not experience a partial paralysis in this stage. The non-rem stage is composed of four sub stages - stage 1 associated with light sleep, stage 2 by true sleep, and stages 3 and 4 with deep sleep. In human adults, the Non-REM sleep comprises about 75% to 80% of the total sleeping time. The stages are as follows:

**Stage 1: Light sleep**

During the "awake" stage, the brain emits alpha waves having a frequency between 8 to 13 Hz. On the onset of the first stage of Non-REM sleep, the brain undergoes a gradual transition during which the intensity of the waves emitted starts decreasing, and reaches between 4 to 7 Hz characterized by the theta waves. This stage may involve slow eye movement, twitches, and even "hypnic jerks" commonly referred to as "sleep start" or "night start" during which the subject awakens suddenly just when he or she is about to fall asleep. The voluntary muscles and metabolic activities start slowing down. The individual can be easily awakened during this stage of sleep.

**Stage 2: True sleep**

Generally within 10 to 15 minutes of the first stage of light sleep, the second stage of true sleep sets in which lasts approximately between 20 to 25 minutes. This second stage of Non-REM sleep is characterized by "sleep spindles" ranging from 11 to 16 Hz during which the brain inhibits various processes to keep the subject in a tranquil state, and the K-complex which suppresses cortical arousal to prevent any external stimuli from signaling danger and aid sleep-based memory consolidation. During this stage, no eye movements occur, and the breathing pattern, as well as the heart rate, slows down. This stage comprises about 45% to 55% of the total sleep consumed by adults.

**Stages 3 and 4: Deep sleep**

During the third stage of Non-REM sleep, the brain starts emitting delta waves having high amplitude (75 µV) and low-frequency (0.5 to 2 Hz). The breathing and heart rates are at their lowest. Parasomnias - a category of sleep disorders associated with abnormal and unnatural body movements, abnormal behavior pattern, uncontrolled emotions, and abnormal perceptions generally occur during this stage. Sleeping disorders such as night terrors, sleepwalking, nocturnal enuresis (bedwetting), and somniloquy (talking aloud in one's sleep) are also associated with this stage. The fourth stage of Non-REM sleep is associated with rhythmic breathing and restricted muscle activity.

**Dreams**

From a scientific point of view, there is no fixed definition of "dreaming". A dream can be interpreted as a succession of images, sounds, and emotions that the human mind experiences during the sleeping process. The basic purpose and manifestation of the dreaming phenomenon are still not clearly understood, and scientists have several hypotheses which try to explain the process. However, it is commonly believed amongst scientists that dreams are basically a result of certain psychological, or neuropsychological activities occurring in a certain portion of the brain. Dreams are associated with the psychological aspect of the brain - the non-tangible part (mind), and not the tangible part (brain). It's important to differentiate between the two. During the lifetime, it is believed a human being spends approximately six years dreaming, which comes to around two hours on a daily basis as an average if we are to consider the average lifespan of a person. It is still unknown exactly how and why dreams originate, and whether there is a single origin, or multiple portions of the brain are involved.

**Difference between REM and Non-REM sleep dreams**

There is a subtle difference between the dreams occurring during the REM and Non-REM stages of sleep. Dreams occurring during the Non-REM stage are brief and fragmentary, do not have any lasting impression on the individual, and they are easily forgotten. In this particular stage, the individual is less likely to experience any lucid and clear visual images resulting out of the dreaming process. During the REM dream stage, a portion of the brain called "pons" shuts off all chemical signals associated with voluntary muscles functioning to the spinal cord. This causes temporary paralysis, and the body becomes incapable of any voluntary movements. The REM sleep signal originates from the pons. This is a natural defense mechanism which prevents the person from harming himself or herself during sleep, since the dreams occurring during the REM stage of sleep can seem to be real and life-like, and this can cause the subject to respond physically in accordance to the particular dream pattern. It is believed pons secretes acetylcholine, a chemical compound that acts as a neurotransmitter, during the REM stage which is transmitted to different parts of the forebrain. This causes cholinergic activation within the affected tissue areas. This is what causes the "dream" phenomenon.

**Biological Rhythm.**

Much of our behavior follows regular rhythms. Daily rhythms in behavior and physiological processes are found throughout the plant and animal world. We have a number of natural cycles, which form part of our everyday lives. Some of these operate over several weeks, such as the human menstrual cycle, while others are much more rapid, such as the human menstrual cycle, while others are much more rapid, such as the cycles involved in digestion and food intake. Some rhythms, called circadian rhythms, are based on the 24hours of the day, and perhaps the most obvious circadian rhythm is the sleep-wake circle we alternate throughout life, between periods of wakefulness and periods of sleeping, human beings, for the most part, tend to be awake during the day and sleep at night-they are diurnal animals. Other animals are awake at night and sleep during the day, they are known as nocturnal animals.

**Sleep Rhythms**

Research on human sleep is usually conducted in a sleep laboratory such laboratories are equipped with machines for taking electrophysiological measurements. Electrodes placed on the scalp monitor the electroencephalogram (EEG): those attached to the chain monitor muscle activity, which is recorded as the electromyogram (EMG) electrodes attached around the eyes monitor eye movements, recorded as electrooculogram (EOG) in addition, other electrodes can be used to monitor autonomic measures such as heart rate electrocardiogram - EKG or ECG respiration electros ethogram-ESC and skin conductance (or galvanic skin response-GSR).

During wakefulness. The EEG of a normal person shows two basic patterns of activity: alpha activity and beta activity. The alpha activity consists of regular, medium frequency waves of 8-12 Hz. the brain produces this activity when a person is resting quietly, not particularly aroused or excited and not engaged in a strenuous mental activity. Alpha waves occur most often when the eyes are closed. The beta activity consists of irregular, mostly low-amplitude waves of 13-30Hz. This activity occurs when a person is alert and attentive to an event in the environment or is thinking activity.

During the course of the night, a normal person passes through four different stages (or levels) of sleep several times. Moving from higher to lower levels of sleep, and back to higher levels again. This cycle is repeated several times during a typical night although the deeper levels of sleep tend to be reached only during the first few cycles. Towards the end of the night, sleep cycles become shallower and the person is liable to wake up easily. These changes in EEG pattern reflect how deeply the person is asleep.

Stage 1: Sleep is marked by the presence of some theta activity (3.5-7.5Hz) the level is actually a transition between sleep and wakefulness. It lasts for about ten minutes. It is the lightest level of sleep from which one can be very easily awakened. Breathing is irregular and the muscles begin to relax as the person transit into the next stage.

Stage 2: The EEG during this stage is generally irregular but contains periods of theta activity sleep spindles and K complexes. Sleep spindles are short burst of waves of about 12-14 Hz that occur between two and five times during stages 1-4 of sleep. They presumably represent the activity of a mechanism that decreases the brain's sensitivity to sensory input and thus keeps the person asleep. The sleep of older people contain fewer sleep spindles and is generally accompanied by more awakenings during the night. K complexes are sudden. Sharp waveforms, which unlike sleep spindles, are usually found only during stage 2 sleep. They spontaneously occur at the rate of approximately one per minute but are often can be triggered by noise. They represent mechanisms involved in keeping the person asleep. Stage 2 sleep lasts for about 15 minutes and is a deeper level of sleep. Persons woken up during this level of sleep will deny having been asleep.

Stage 3: Sleep is marked by the occurrence of high-amplitude delta activity (less than 3.5 Hz). this is a transition from the light sleep of stages 1 and 2 to a deeper sleep. The distinction between stage 3 and stage 4 is not clear-cut; stage 3 contains 20-50 percent delta activity: and stage 4 contains more than 50 percent. Stage 3 sleep last for about 20 minutes.

Stage 4 Sleep is the deepest level of sleep from which it is difficult to awaken the sleeper. It is characterized; also, by delta activity (EEG readings of less than 2.5 Hz) usually takes more than half an hour to reach this level of sleep. About 90 minutes after the beginning of sleep (and about 45 minutes after the onset of stage 4 sleep) they will be an abrupt change in a number of the physiological measures being taken. The EEG recording becomes desynchronized (i.e. irregular, with a sprinkling of theta waves. Very similar to the record obtained during stage 1 sleep. The EOG will record that the eyes are rapidly darting back and forth beneath the eye, the EMG becomes silent due to a profound loss of muscle tonus. Thus apart from an occasional twitching of some muscles, the person is actually paralyzed during this period. This peculiar stage of sleep is quite distinct from the quiet sleep we saw earlier. This type of sleep is usually referred to as REM or rapid eye movement sleep. It has also been called paradoxical sleep because of the presence of beta activity. This is usually seen during wakefulness or stage sleep.

REM Sleep Stages 1-4 are usually referred to as non-REM or quiet sleep (QS). Stages 3 and 4 are referred to as slow-wave sleep or deep quiet sleep (DQS): while stages 1 and 2 are known as light quiet sleep (LQS).

On the average, most normal persons have four or five periods of active sleep at night. Each of these cycles lasts for about 90 minutes, containing a 20- 30 minutes about of REM as sleep.

# Children and Sleep

Healthy sleep patterns are important for people of any age. However, when it comes to kids, instilling the right habits in them from the start can save them and you a whole host of future problems. Sleep is of vital importance for all of us, but it is particularly so for growing babies and children. Making sure that your kids get the sleep they need is an extremely important part of parenting.

Sleeping is one of the most important and pleasant activities of human life. Waking up feeling refreshed makes the whole day much better. It is vital for our health, mental, emotional and physical. Circadian rhythms are regulated by the light and dark, however, these rhythms actually take time to develop. Usually, by six weeks old babies are beginning to develop such sleep-wake cycles.

It has been shown that by the age of two, most children have actually spent more time asleep than awake. Most kids will spend about forty percent of their childhood asleep. Babies, spend about fifty percent of their time in each of the states of sleep REM and non -REM. By about six months of age, REM sleep accounts for approximately thirty percent of sleep.

Newborns sleep on average a total of 10-18 hours of the day sleeping. These sleeping periods may range from only a few seconds to a number of hours at a time. The sleep of newborns is interspersed by their need to be changed, nurtured and fed. But even at this early stage developing good sleep patterns is essential.

Babies should be put down while they are sleepy rather than once they are asleep. In this way, experts say that they will learn to fall asleep better on their own. As a parent, being aware of your baby's sleep signals is very important.

Some baby's rub their eyes, while others might fuss or cry. These signals will let you know that they should be ready for a nap. Another important point is to help them get used to the circadian rhythms by keeping them more awake during the day with light and some noise and making nighttime dark and quiet. This can help encourage night time sleeping.

For infants from 3-11 months, nighttime feedings may become increasingly unnecessary. By 9 months, seventy-eight percent of infants will be able to sleep through the night. Naps will become less frequent throughout the day as well. Again putting infants to bed when they are drowsy will help them become self-soothers. Developing regular daytime and bedtime schedules will help ease the transition as well being consistent about these routines. Making the sleep environment as friendly as possible for the infant will also go a long way to helping with sleep.

From ages one to three, kids need about 12-14 hours of sleep a day. One nap a day lasting about one to three hours for those aged 18 months or older is fine, but these should not occur too close to bedtime. Many toddlers do experience some sleep troubles at this stage including separation anxiety, night fears, and/or getting out of bed as part of their newfound independence. Some tips to help deal with these issues include: making the bedroom environment the same every night including the bedtime schedule. Setting limits that are consistent and encouraging the use of a security object, be it a blanket or stuffed animal.

Once your child is a preschooler, from age 3-5, they will typically need between 11 and 13 hours per night. Children at this stage may still be experiencing nighttime fears and thus may be having trouble sleeping.

The same principles here also apply. Consistency, friendly environment, and security all help establish good habits. As your child gets older you will be able to explain in more detail the importance of sleep and of regular sleeping schedules for their health and wellbeing.

Once a child reaches the prepubescent years, TV, video games, internet and other media, as well as caffeinated beverages all, may contribute to sleep disorders. Making sure that a calm, cool and dark environment is available and that TV and other such media is limited especially before bed will all help your child achieve a better night's rest.

Teenagers need a great deal more sleep than adults do. As we get older we need less and less sleep. According to the American Sleep Disorders Association, teenagers on average need about nine and a half hours of sleep a night. Most interestingly, researchers have found that teenagers need about two hours more sleep a night than their siblings of eight to ten years. This is in contradiction however to how parents usually organize sleep routines. Parents most often allow their teenagers to stay up later than younger siblings.

Because of the growth rate and hormonal changes occurring among teenagers, more sleep is needed. A lack of sleep at this juncture can result in a variety of ill effects. Poor school performance and mood changes can be just some of the most immediate consequences. Car accidents and depression can also be contributed to by poor sleep habits.

In order to tell if your teenager is not getting enough sleep, you can check for some common symptoms. Is your teen having difficulty getting up in the morning? Is he or she irritable in the afternoons? Does your teen fall asleep during the day or oversleep on weekends? Does he or she wake up during the night and have trouble getting back to sleep?

If you've answered yes to some of these questions then your teenager might not be getting enough sleep. Be sure to follow some of the guidelines listed above and/or talk to your health care professional about how to start instituting better sleep regimes.

By following these guidelines early on you will have a better chance of preventing later sleep disturbances.

Good sleep habits begin at a very early age. If you are just starting out though remember the above suggestions. Teens taught about healthy sleep patterns. Beginning a discussion with your child about the benefits of sleep will help them understand why you might be implementing some of the less well-received rules. For instance, if you explain to your child that engaging with media right before bed can have a negative consequence on proper sleep, then he or she might be more inclined to obey such suggestions.

As with younger children, sleeping spaces should be dark, quiet and inviting. Comfortable beds and a good room temperature are also important. Following a regular schedule rather than trying to make up for lost sleep on weekends is also important. All of these solutions will help children of all ages develop healthy sleep habits. We can't live without sleep, so make it is well worth the effort to make sure that your children are getting enough.

# Types of Sleep Disorders

**Insomnia**

The most frequently found sleeping disorder in youngsters is insomnia, which is indicated by the problems in going to sleep. Regularly caused by hysteria and depression, this condition also makes it difficult for an individual to stay in the state of sleep for lengthy periods, so giving the individual low quality sleep. Short-term insomnia can be due to nerve-wrangling circumstances like a sickness, stress while at work, college or social circle or any other exhausting events happening in one's life. Lingering insomnia from another perspective includes sleep turmoil for a minimum of 3 months.

**Sleep Apnea**

In sleep apnea, your respiring stops or gets awfully shallow while you are sleeping. Each pause in breathing usually lasts 10-20 seconds or even more, and the pauses can happen twenty to thirty times or even more an hour. In the episodes of apnea, the sleeper wakes up to respire again, interrupting sleep and also is affected with a temporary shortage of oxygen.

Symptoms of Sleep Apnea include:

* Frequent gaps in respiring while asleep (apnea)

* Gasping or choking for air to restart respiring, regularly causing sleeper or partner to wake

* Loud snoring

* Feeling unrefreshed after a night's sleep and unnecessary daytime weariness

The most typical type of sleep apnea is obstructive sleep apnea. Factors behind sleep apnea are typically physical in nature, including additional weight or tissue (occasionally from being obese or fat), enormous tonsils or adenoids, sinus congestion or blockage or a singular formed head, neck or jaw.

CPAP, a mechanical device worn while sleeping which supplies continual air pressure to keep the airway open, is the most commended treatment for moderate to severe sleep apnea.

CPAP can take a little getting used to but provides effective relief when used in the right way.

Self-help treatments, like shedding pounds, elevating the head of the bed or sleeping on your side, may also be effective cures for mild sleep apnea. Dental appliances and surgery are also treatment choices.

**Snoring**

Snoring, which is often confused with sleep apnea, could be a major barrier to quality sleep both for yourself and your better half.

Snoring is due to a narrowing of your airway, either from poor sleep posture, excess weight or physical disorders of your throat. A narrow airway gets in the way of smooth respiring and creates the sound of snoring.

There are many self-help cures and cures for snoring. If you're a mild snorer, sleeping on your side, raising the head of your bed, or shedding weight may stop the snoring. Do not give up attempting to find a solution for your snoring it'll make you and your better half sleep sounder.

Restless Legs Syndrome (RLS) and Periodic Limb Movements in Sleep (PLMS).

The desire to move occurs when resting or lying down and is mostly due to uncomfortable, tingly, or creeping sensations in the legs or influenced limbs. Movement lightens the feelings, but only for a bit.

Periodic Limb Movement Disorder ( PLMD ) is a related condition concerning involuntary, rhythmical limb movements, either while asleep or when awake. While the majority who've Twitchy Legs Syndrome also have PLMD, only some individuals with PLMD also have RLS.

RLS may run in families.

Alternative cures, life changes, and even nutritive additions have proved useful for RLS and PLMD sufferers.

**Narcolepsy**

Narcolepsy is a neurological disorder that causes acute sleepiness and can even make somebody go to sleep all of a sudden and without any warning.

The sleep attacks experienced by folks with narcolepsy happen even after getting plenty of sleep at night and make it hard for folk to live ordinary lives. Dropping off during activities like walking, driving or working can have dangerous results.

* Discontinuous, uncontrollable episodes of dropping off in the daytime

* Exaggerated daytime sleepiness

* Sudden, fugitive loss of muscle control during emotional situations (cataplexy)

Treatment needs a mix of medication, behavior treatments, and support.

**REM sleep behavior disorder**

REM sleep behavior disorder causes interruptions in the brain during REM sleep. During REM ( i.e, the dream part of sleep ), an area of the brainstem called the pons sends signals to the cerebral cortex, which is the area of the brain answerable for thinking and organizing info. The pons also sends signals to muscles in the body during REM, causing a kind of brief paralysis.

In somebody with REM sleep behavior disorder, these signals transliterate into pictures that make up dreams. If the signals are meddled with, the individual may physically act out dreams while sleeping.

Cataplexy is weakness or paralysis of the muscles. In narcoleptic patients, it could be caused by exhaustion and intense emotions and can be accompanied by short, sudden episodes of laughter or outrage.

When cataplexy happens, people who are standing may fall down.

**Sleep Paralysis**

Sleep paralysis is the incapacity to move the arms, legs, or whole body that happens when somebody is going to sleep or awakening. It typically lasts a particularly temporary time period. Folk who experience sleep paralysis may become extraordinarily concerned and frequently regain movement only if they hear an intense noise or another impulse.

**Jet lag**

Jet lag is a physiological condition which is a consequence of modifications to circadian rhythms; it is assessed as one of the circadian rhythm sleep disorders.

**Circadian rhythm sleep disorder**

Examples include jet lag and shift work sleep disorder. Sufferers aren't able to wake and sleep in the standard routines needed to function in standard work, college and social settings.

**Delayed sleep-phase syndrome**

Delayed sleep phase syndrome is a circadian rhythm sleep problem, a protracted disorder chronic disorder of the timing of sleep, top period of alertness, core body temperature, hormonal and other daily rhythms relative to societal norms.

# What Women Need To Know About Sleep Disorders

**Women and sleep problems**

There is sufficient research to show that women are more prone to sleep-related disorders than men. One of the main reasons for this is the hormonal make-up of a lady. When there is a spike or a drop in hormone levels, especially during the menstrual cycle, pre or post pregnancy and at the time of menopause, women are found to report more sleep-related issues than men. In fact, women are 1.4 times more likely to complain of insomnia than men would. Also, sometimes, the problem women have is excessive sleeping and sleepiness.

There is no racial basis on which sleep disorders affect women, but their side effects are plenty. There is an increased chance of stroke as well as cardiac trouble in women. Hypertension and obesity are also possible. Since sleep controls most of our bodily functions, there is every chance of lack of sleep being harmful to our health.

Research has shown that younger women tend to sleep better compared to older women. In some cases, it is seen that women in their reproductive years continue to have sleep-related issues. There are quite a few factors that influence sleep patterns in a woman. Some of them are:

**Factors that influence sleep patterns in women**

**Hormonal changes** - Hormonal changes during the menstrual cycle also cause insomnia or even daytime sleepiness. Besides having direct or indirect effects on sleep, they can also affect moods and emotions. This is commonly known as premenstrual stress, and almost 80% of women report having it.

**Pregnancy** - Pregnancy can also affect sleep patterns. Usually, it is noticed that in the first trimester, women need more sleep and more so during the daytime. During the second trimester, this changes and sleep patterns are more comfortable. Most of the third-trimester women suffer from lack of sleep due to discomfort, acidity, a constant need to urinate, heartburn and fetal movements at odd times. Even pain in the lower back tends to keep women up. Sometimes, there is swelling in the nasal passage resulting in sleep apnea or snoring.

**Menstruation and menopause-related causes**: Menopause and women aging can result in both physical and hormonal changes, and this can cause sleep-related trouble. There is a tendency to remain awake at night and be restless during the day. Menopausal women also suffer from hot flashes and night sweats, and this is an indication of lower estrogen levels. Deep sleep remains elusive at this time and being awake at night a constant.

**Insomnia Among Women**

Insomnia is the most widely reported sleep disorder in women followed by fluctuating sleep patterns, stress, daytime sleepiness and the inability to wake up on time. Psychological stress can be one of the triggers as well. This is especially seen in working mothers who tend to ignore fatigue and other such symptoms that can lead to sleep-related trouble in the long run. Insomnia in women can include the inability to fall asleep, get deep sleep or rising too soon. Many also find it difficult to go back to sleep once awake.

Menopausal women tend to suffer from sleep-disordered breathing. This results in loud snoring and interrupted deep sleep. Most women are unable to go back to sleep and are often tired in the daytime. This is a time when sleep apnea sets in for women beyond 50 years of age.

Women can also suffer from restless leg syndrome (RLS) or the periodic limb movement disorder (PLMD). Both can be very disturbing to sound sleep. The real causes for these conditions are not really known. RLS tends to set in just before a person goes to sleep and is a constant strain on the calves. This strain can be relieved by movement, something that happens rather involuntarily at times. PLMD results in periodic movements of the leg that tend to awaken someone. It is also a cause of insomnia. It has an opposite effect at times where it causes excessive sleep. Both of these conditions are commonly seen in senior citizens.

Excessive sleepiness in the daytime is known as narcolepsy. It is characterized by sleep attacks and what is known as cataplexy. A sleep attack is where there is an uncontrollable urge to go to sleep whereas cataplexy is characterized by a sudden loss of muscle tone before which a person will have an unwarranted emotional episode. Sleep paralysis and hypnagogic hallucinations also occur on occasion.

Women today tend to deal with multiple roles at a given time -- professional, wife, mother, caregiver and more. Often with reduced times for themselves and extreme levels of stress, sleep deprivation is a natural result. Erratic work and lifestyles tend to lead to sleeping trouble as well, which is further accented when faced with hormonal imbalance.

Many women find it comforting to take in some caffeine or nicotine closer to bedtime. However, these are stimulants and often don't help to induce sound sleep. The same goes with vices like alcohol that can lead to fragmented sleep and nightmares. It is often seen that sleep disorders are common among older women.

Being overweight puts a woman at risk for sleep disorders. Following are the three disorders common to women who are overweight. In many cases, the symptoms tend to overlap.

**Sleep Risk Factors from Being Overweight**

Inability to fall asleep: Often this is seen in younger women who are overweight, and it is directly related to an unhealthy lifestyle and a much-stressed existence.

Inability to remain asleep: Constantly being roused from sleep for a range of reasons also occur among those who are overweight. Other health-related reasons may be the last trimester of pregnancy, chronic arthritis and the possible intake of pain medication.

Constant daytime sleepiness: Most menopausal women suffer from excessive sleepiness in the daytime. Sometimes nasal passages tend to get blocked, and this results in loud snoring that further acts as a deterrent to good sleep.

When it comes to women and sleep problems, there is a range of reasons why women suffer. In many cases, it is the natural order of things based on the hormonal condition of the woman. Recognizing the symptoms and getting prompt help from a specialist can reduce the symptoms.

# Medical Problems and Sleeping Too Much

When it comes to sleep, like anything else in life, has been reported that moderation is key for good health and long life. Sleeping too little causes health problems, but did you know that sleeping too much can cause the same or more medicals problems such as diabetes and heart disease and is linked to weight gain, Parkinson's and depression? Are you sleeping too much? Researchers do point out that the amount of sleep varies with age and that people that are stressed or sick will tend to sleep more. Other factors that cause oversleeping are those that have less access to health care which may have undiagnosed mental and physical illnesses such as heart disease and depression. People that abuse alcohol and drugs are inclined to oversleep. Then there are those that just love to sleep or at least like to take a nap in the afternoon.

The National Sleep Foundation recommends that adults should get around seven to nine hours of sleep a night. Some research has found that long sleep duration of nine hours or more is associated with illness and death. What medical problems cause people to sleep too much?

Hypersomnia is a medical disorder that causes people to experience extreme sleepiness during the day which is not relieved by napping. People with hypersomnia crave sleep and can suffer from anxiety, low energy and lack of concentration. They not only sleep at various times during the day, they also sleep for long periods during the night. Causes of hypersomnia are brain damage, clinical depression, uremia, obesity, and fibromyalgia. Symptoms are like those with other sleep disorders such as narcolepsy, sleep apnea and restless legs syndrome (RLS). Some people get hypersomnia as a result of drug or alcohol abuse, drug or alcohol withdrawal or as a drug side effect as with some psychotropics for depression, anxiety or bipolar disorder.

Kleine-Levin Syndrome (aka Sleeping Beauty Sickness) is the most recognized form of recurrent hypersomnia, though it is very rare, these people often sleep up to eighteen hours a day and yet do not feel refreshed upon waking. Patients that suffer from Kleine-Levin Syndrome only wake up to go to the bathroom and eat. When they are awake they tend to be confused, lethargic and are indifferent to the world around them. Many cannot go to school, work or even care for themselves. The cause of Kleine-Levin is unknown. This disorder affects teens more than adults and in many cases disappears as mysteriously as it appears; often when patients reach their twenties.

Non-insulin dependent (type 2) Diabetes has been linked to those that sleep more than nine hours and less than five hours a night by a risk greater than 50% as a result of a study of almost 9,000 Americans. It is not known why longer sleep durations contribute to diabetes, although increased time asleep to compensate for lack of sleep is one possible reason. There are more studies needed to determine if longer sleep periods actually worsen the metabolic syndrome which is a cluster of risk factors including high blood pressure, obesity, and insulin resistance which contribute to heart disease and stroke.

Obesity affects those that sleep too little as well as those that sleep nine to ten hours a night. According to a report, 21% of those monitored over a six-year period were more likely overweight when sleeping too much than those that slept seven to eight hours even when taking in to account caloric intake and exercise. In another measure, nearly half of those who slept nine hours or more each night were physically inactive during the day, which was associated with other health issues that make exercise more difficult.

Headaches and Back Pain and other minor illnesses cause people to sleep more than usual. But did you know that oversleeping causes headaches? When you oversleep your brain produces more serotonin a hormone that affects our neurotransmitters causing a headache in the morning. Too much time in bed can cause stiffness resulting in back pain. It is not only important for you to have the right mattress for your back you also need to keep a regular exercise program to keep the weight off and not lay down longer than seven to eight hours. The longer you stay in bed, the longer it will take your back to adjust to your redistributed weight and stiffness upon standing.

Mental Illness is associated with irregular sleeping habits. Depression can worsen when you oversleep and it is important to maintain regular sleeping habits to recover. SAD or seasonal affective disorder is a condition where your brain produces too much melatonin because there aren't enough daylight hours which causes people to sleep longer and take naps in the afternoon. SAD triggers feelings of despair, misery, guilt, hopelessness or anxiety. You may find normal tasks become frustratingly difficult, you may cry for no apparent reason or be unable to concentrate. Exercise, taking Vitamin D and light therapy help those that suffer from SAD.

Cardiovascular diseases are 38% more likely to happen for those that sleep nine to 11 hours a night according to a report by The Nurses' Health Study involving nearly 72,000 women than those that slept seven to eight hours. With ten hours' sleep, the death rate from a heart attack or stroke for women over 70 increased 167%, while for men aged 50 to 59, it increased by 286%. Researchers have not yet identified a reason for the connection between oversleeping and heart disease as the evidence does not show which came first-the arterial disease, or the tendency to sleep longer than average.

Parkinson's is more probable or twice as likely to develop for those people that sleep at least nine hours versus those that sleep on six hours or less. A study was done by the National Institute of Health, a U.S. government body studies 80,000 nurses over 24 years and found that those that slept eight hours were 60% prone to the disease while only 10% for those that slept seven. The most at risk were those that slept at least nine hours a night or 80%. At the end of the study 181 developed Parkinson's.

What they did find interesting was that night-shift workers had lower levels of the hormones melatonin and estradiol. Some scientists believe higher levels contribute to the development of Parkinson's and a need to sleep may be an early sign of the condition. Other symptoms include tremors, stiffness and a gradual slowing down of the body. Further research is needed to make a final conclusion on how sleep is related to Parkinson's.

It's a matter of life and death as studies show us that people who sleep nine hours or more have higher death rates than those that sleep seven to eight hours a night. If you feel you are sleeping too much consult with your doctor as he may recommend a further test to determine why you oversleep, as too much sleep can be an underlying medical condition.

# Basic Rules for Better Sleep

Millions of people have trouble sleeping. It's estimated, in fact, that ten percent of Americans suffer from insomnia at any given time, and as a result, millions of sleeping pills are consumed every night. There are, however, several things you can do that will significantly improve your sleep, and surprisingly, many of the people who suffer from insomnia never use them. It's well-known that sleep is affected by both physiological (body) and psychological (mind) factors, and both must be addressed if you are to improve your sleep.

The body factors are related to what is called the "body clock." In reality, there are several body clocks. One is related directly to sleep; several others are indirectly related in that they regulate the hormones that your body gives off at night such as melatonin, serotonin, growth hormone and cortisol. A clock also regulates your body temperature throughout the night. Under ideal circumstances, these clocks are all synchronized.

The psychological or mind factors that affect your sleep are your thought, emotions, anxieties, stress and so on. They are usually associated with an overactive mind, and people with insomnia have been shown to have overactive minds; in particular, their minds are cluttered with anxious thoughts that create negative emotions and stresses that don't allow them to sleep. You have to control both your body clock and your thought if you want a good nights sleep. Five rules that will help you do this are as follows:

1. **Start by re-setting (or re-aligning) your body clock.**

Your body clock is like an ordinary clock in that it has a period of 24 hours, and like ordinary clocks, it can get out of aligning. What does this mean? Your body clock adjusts to your schedule of sleep and wakefulness, and because it knows this schedule, it tells your body when to get ready for bed, and when to rise in the morning. As long as you keep a regular schedule, this clock will operate effectively. But if you stay up late and begin sleeping in, particularly on weekends, your body clock can't adjust properly, and you find you aren't sleeping when you're supposed to be or waking up before you normally do. In short, your body clock has been knocked out of adjustment and needs to be re-set.

Furthermore, your body clock controls your body temperature at night. It allows it to decrease by one or two degrees until about 4: oo A.M. then it begins to rise slowly. About two hours later it gives you a wake-up call. If your bedtime and rise time are irregular, this clock is not sure when to wake you. So you have to re-set it by getting back to a regular schedule.

**2. Once your body clock is reset, you have to develop sufficient sleep drive, which in turn creates a sleep "pressure" that puts you to sleep.**

You create a sleep drive by creating a "sleep debt." Most people stay awake approximately 16 out of the 24 hours of the day. This means they have an 8-hour sleep debt when they go to bed. If you're having problems sleeping, however, an 8-hour sleep debt may not be enough to put you to sleep quickly. Your sleep debt, which creates your sleep drive, is increased by staying awake and active as long as possible during the day. In particular, make sure you get as much sunlight as possible (it's sunlight that builds up your sleep drive). Also, you should not nap during the day (assuming you have insomnia), and you should make sure you don't sleep in to make up for sleep you may have lost during the night. If you lost some sleep (assuming you don't sleep in) your sleep drive will be greater the next night because you'll have a larger sleep debt. This will create extra "pressure' for you to sleep.

**3. Make sure you "prepare" yourself for sleep**

Many people are tense and have anxious thoughts throughout the day (mostly because of our fast, high-pressure, society, and they have trouble relaxing before they go to bed. Their mind is in "full gear" all day long and they are unable to shut it down before they go to bed.

It's important, however, to make sure you "let go" before you go to bed. There are usually two types of thoughts in their minds: non-emotional and emotional. The worst is the emotional thoughts, but non-emotional (decisions, planning for the next day) thoughts can also be a problem. It's important to allow for a "cool down" period before you go to bed to get rid of them. This means you should spend at least half-an-hour (or preferably, an hour) relaxing and preparing yourself for sleep. Several of the things you can do during this time is:

*read

*watch TV (make sure it is nonviolent)

*take a warm bath

*Meditate

Make sure your mind is "quiet" before you go to bed. Also, you should make sure you are sleepy. If you're not sleepy, wait until you are.

## 4. Once in bed, don't try to force yourself to sleep

The object, once you are in bed is to allow yourself to go to sleep as quickly as possible. If you are awake for a half-hour or longer don't fall into the trap of trying to force yourself to sleep. This is, in fact, the worst thing you can do. Think about when you were younger and slept well. Did you go to bed and "try to sleep?" No, sleep just came -- usually with no effort. So don't try to force yourself to sleep -- let it come naturally. This may seem like it is easier said than done. But if your sleep drive is well-primed and you have a good sleep debt, you will sleep. If you're still awake after an hour or so, get up, go to another room and read or meditate until you are sleepy.

## 5. Quiet your mind

If you are still having problems, you will have to quiet your mind further, and there are a couple of different approaches to this. The first thing is to completely clear your mind -- make it blank. Then think of an enjoyable image: a mountain scene you once saw, an enjoyable day at the beach, or a family gathering. Keep your mind fixed on it. Relax and enjoy it until you fall asleep.

Finally, don't worry if you don't get 7 or 8 hours of sleep. Any sleep you lose will help build up a better sleep drive for the following night. And don't worry if you wake up in the night. Accept it, relax, roll over and go back to sleep.

# **Stress Relief Solution: Sleep**

If you are looking for stress relief- look no further than your bed and your pillow! You must have the proper amount and type of sleep if you really want to manage your stress!

A poll taken by the National Sleep Foundation found that sleep debt is a problem for more than half of America's workforce. Their data suggests that in the last century we've reduced the average amount of time we sleep by 20 percent.

Of course, I suppose that most of us recognize that if we don't get adequate sleep for a night or two, we may not function as well the next day. If we work a job where accuracy is super important, or if we are driving a long distance, we sure don't want to be sleepy. And we may even realize that adequate sleep affects our immune system. With a lack of sleep, we may be more likely to get sick. But tying the optimum amount of sleep into various diseases and even our longevity...well, maybe that is food for thought!

In reality, sleep deprivation is taking a serious toll on our overall health! In Super Foods Health style by Steven G Pratt, he reports that a sleep debt of merely 3 or 4 hours in a week may have a direct bearing on the following:

• Obesity

• Coronary heart disease

• Hypertension

• Diabetes

• Immune function

• Cognitive performance

• Longevity

Sleep deprivation is a stressor and when you don't get enough sleep, your glucocorticoids go up which are the main hormone groups that cause the stress response in your body. The group of stress hormones that are released during the stress response are called glucocorticoids and include norepinephrine, adrenaline, and a variety of other hormones designed to make you very alert.

If these glucocorticoid levels go up they can actually inhibit your ability to sleep. In other words, not getting enough sleep triggers the hormones that will make it difficult for you to sleep! The good news is that if you are exhausted enough, you will sleep anyway- but even then, the quality of your sleep will be affected by these hormones.

Lose sleep- Die Young!

You do not have to lose huge amounts of sleep before it takes a toll. One study found that sleeping less than 4 hours per night was associated with a 2.8 times higher rate of mortality for men and a 1.5 times higher rate for women. The author of this study also found that length of sleep time was a better predictor of mortality than smoking, cardiac disease, or hypertension.

Another study found that people who slept six hours or less a night had a 70 percent higher mortality rate over a nine-year period than those who slept seven to eight hours a night!

More important than how much sleep we get, is the type of sleep that we get. Although there are several different stages of sleep, the most important is call REM or Rapid Eye Movement sleep. During this stage of sleep, the secondary sensory cortex becomes active- which is a major processing center of the brain. This is where we process information without having a visual or auditory stimulation. We call this dreaming.

**What Really Happens When I'm Dreaming?**

In the 1970's there were extensive sleep studies at Berkeley University in California. It was through these studies and subsequent studies that we discovered the stages of sleep, what they all do, and what happens when you don't get them!

During dreaming, many different parts of our brain including the limbic system, the emotional part of our brains, is highly active and seems to be processing emotions from the day.

As a Master Rapid Eye Therapist, I certainly understand the importance of this process. In fact, Rapid Eye Therapy harnesses the power REM to by putting a person into the same brain wave patterns found in the brain during REM so that we can quickly and easily process both conscious and unconscious emotions! (See the Managing Your Emotions section for more information.)

We could say, that when you are missing sleep, you are missing the chance to literally process the emotions of your day- it's like having your own therapy session every night! In fact, during the REM stage of sleep, the eyes blink rapidly, but the eyeballs actually move around in various positions that cause certain parts of the brain to fire in the following sequence:

* As you look off to the right or left, the auditory part of the brain fires- processing everything you might have HEARD,

* The eyes move up to the left- and the Memory centers of the brain fire processing MEMORIES

* The eyes look straight up causing the visual cortex to fire, processing everything you have SEEN.

* The eyes then look up and to the right, firing the area of the brain that runs your habitual PATTERNS.

* Then the eyes look straight down, which fires the limbic areas of the brain-processing all the emotions-- everything you FELT.

This process is what I call a "body google" -- searching for all the stressful events that are overloading your body and brain! This process keeps repeating for about 20 minutes, all the while you are dreaming. It would appear that the body is literally designed to process the stress of the day, especially when you see what happens next!

At the end of all the blinking and eye rolling, something very strange happens. The eyes roll back in the head, and there is a literal "gas "of negatively charged ions that come out of the eyes! WHAT THE???? It would appear that after all this "googling" that the "residue" of all that stress from the day comes out of your body in the form of negatively charged ions! That happens to you every night and it should happen three times a night --if you are getting enough sleep!

Who would have thought when you sleep you are really working on your "issues" and processing all the things that give you stress! The scary thing is that many sleeping pills, like the popular Ambien, actually inhibit you from ever going into REM stage of sleep! You are missing out on a huge benefit of sleep!

In fact, in subsequent studies, it was found that conditions like post-partum depression may be caused from the mother being awakened so many times with the baby during the night that they never get any REM stage sleep. This is thought to be a major cause of depression /anxiety in new mothers.

The glucocorticoid hormones that are released during stress can also make it not only difficult to go to sleep, but also interrupt the REM stage of sleep.

It is clear that all the stages of sleep have a purpose and that missing REM sleep stages, or not getting enough of them by not sleeping long enough can have dangerous consequences

**How Much Sleep Do We Need?**

In order to get experience REM three times a night, and all the stages of sleep you need to really have optimum performance and prevent the stress response in the body, the following guidelines are suggested:

• A six to twelve-year-old will need between 10 ½ and 11 ½ hours of sleep a night.

• A teenager will require a little less sleep, probably around 9 or 10 hours a night.

• An adult should be getting 7 to 8 hours sleep each night.

In addition, it is better for you to sleep at night than during the daytime. In fact, sleeping between the hours of 10 P.M. and 6 A.M. is considered to be optimal. This allows for your body to restore its needed melatonin levels in a natural way.

**Create a Peaceful Environment**

The environment around you absolutely has an effect on your ability to relax and go to sleep. Here are some suggestions for creating a peaceful environment, taken from my experience with Feng Shui:

**• Don't put your bed directly under a window**

Try to avoid this arrangement- as the energy from outside cascades down on you all night If you have to sleep under a window, put a heavy drape over the window and keep it closed at night.

**• Get rid of the lights**

Even a bright alarm clock can trigger your pineal gland that it's time to wake up instead of going to sleep! Cover up all offending lights that won't turn off and notice how much better and LONGER you can sleep! Drape your windows if the sun comes in too early in the morning as well.

**• NEVER put a TV /office equipment in your bedroom**

The EMF's (Electric Magnetic Frequencies) from this equipment will disrupt your sleep (not to mention your love life!). Just because you can't see it does not mean it isn't real, and EMF's are real. Sometimes this is unavoidable-- but just realize that this will cause a sleep disruption and if you can, put the TV and offices in other places than the bedroom.

### • Don't sleep directly across from a mirror

Believe it or not, you can actually see with your eyes closed, and seeing an image of what could appear to be another uninvited person in the room can invoke anxiety-- even when you are asleep! Crazy but true!

### • Make your bed-clean up the clutter!

Your mother was right! Getting into a clean fresh made bed can have a very calming effect on your body. Making the bed also keeps animals and unwanted dust and energy off your sheets. Close your drawers, pick up your clothes and you will get an added measure of calm and peaceful rest.

### Your Body's Natural Sleeping Pill

We have talked about how prescription Sleeping pills inhibit REM Sleep and may actually do more harm than good. So what can you do if you can't sleep? Get your body back in balance by turning to Mother Nature!

Melatonin is a natural hormone made by your body's pineal gland. During the day the pineal is inactive, but when darkness comes, the pineal is turned on and begins to actively produce melatonin. In order to get enough melatonin:

1. Get a full night sleep in complete darkness (Get some "Blinders" if you have a lot of bleed-through light in your room

2. Take a Melatonin Producing supplement-

So, close your eyes at night to avoid diabetes, to lose weight, to strengthen your immune system, to feel better, and to live longer!

ACTION ITEM

• Make a commitment to get to bed by 10:00 pm.

• Choose one thing that you could change about your sleeping environment from the list.

• Take an Amino Acid/supplement Based Sleep Aid like Take a Magnesium/Calcium Supplement like CALM

# How to Sleep Better

This is a list of what I believe are the ten most important things anyone can do to improve their sleep. Whether it`s an occasional couple of nights of restless sleep or if it`s full-blown insomnia, these tips helped me and other people I know tremendously.

In order of importance, with 1) being the most important, I urge you to follow these tips and your sleep WILL improve.

Here they are:

1) **Do not take naps in the day.**

The number one most important thing you can do to improve sleep in my experience is NEVER nap or sleep in the day, no matter how tired you are. If you`re very tired it may be a real struggle at first but it WILL pay off and it will get easier.

The reason you shouldn`t nap is that if you`re struggling for sleep we need to quickly reset your Circadian rhythm, and the best way to do this I've found is to avoid daily napping. If you keep napping, it will just delay this resetting from happening and prolong your sleep problems. This is the first part of resetting your Circadian rhythm. Follow this step before moving onto step 2.

2) **Wake up earlier than usual.**

The second part in resetting your Circadian rhythm is setting your alarm to wake you up earlier than usual. Even waking up as little as half an hour earlier than you are used to will make a big difference to readjusting your sleep pattern. Half an hour is the minimum. Try for an hour if you can. This is also a very important step in starting to get a healthy, refreshing night's sleep every night.

The reason this works well is because if the body is used to catching up on sleep later in the morning it doesn't prepare properly for sleep at night. It`s hard to control when you go to sleep, but you can control when you wake up. When you change the time you wake, you can more easily change the whole of your sleep cycle. Set your alarm half hour to one hour earlier.

**3) Do not do anything else in bed apart from sleep and have sex.**

Doing activities such as reading, watching TV, playing games, talking on the phone and eating should all be banned from bed. Only sleep and sex from now on should take place in bed. If you want to read, then find a comfortable chair, if you want to watch TV, sit in the living room (I've banished my TV from my bedroom).

This technique utilizes a simple school of psychology known as Behaviourism. You need to build associations between bed and sleep, not bed and excitement or tension from other activities. Whatever you do in bed, your subconscious will associate that with being in bed.

For example, if you watch horror films in bed, each time you get into bed your subconscious will be thinking about horror films, and the excitement and fear that comes with it. Therefore your heart rate will increase and your mind will find it hard to relax. That`s not a good way to prepare for sleep. Admittedly that is a slightly over the top example but it shows the power of Behaviourism.

**4) Hide the clock.**

It`s simple really, when you know you can`t sleep, and keep reminding yourself you can`t sleep, it becomes stressful, especially if you have an early start. So do yourself a favor and get rid of the glow in the dark alarm clock, move your phone to somewhere else in the room if you use it for an alarm, and get rid of the cuckoo clock, they're old-fashioned and annoying anyway!

**5) Exercise regularly.**

Regular exercise will improve many of the bodies functions such as blood pressure, heart rate, building bone and muscle, combating stress, relieving muscle tension etc. The type of exercise and time of day you do it is important. Afternoon exercise appears to be the most beneficial and it certainly ties in with my own experience. I like to get to sleep around midnight, so I find exercising between 2:00 PM - 4:00 PM is most beneficial.

Exercising late in the evening is not a good idea. I find it hard to wind down after an intense workout. If you must exercise in the evening because of certain commitments I would advise that you exercise at least three hours before your bedtime. This should give you enough time to wind down.

Some researchers believe cardiovascular exercise is best for sleep, which they may be right. I personally like to lift weights, so usually finish off my lifting routine with 15 minutes of moderate cardio and on non-lifting days, I`ll do straight cardio at a higher intensity. This seems to have the most sleep benefits for me as well as the other all round health benefits.

## 6) If you can`t sleep, get up and do something really boring.

This is one tip that I hate, because whenever I can`t do something, like most people I want to try harder, but when it comes to sleep, consciously trying harder to sleep is counterproductive as we all know - most of us from our own experiences.

So, the best thing to do is get up, turn the light on, and do something boring for 15 minutes. This doesn't include watching TV, checking email, exercise, etc. It MUST be boring, an example would be reorganizing your sock drawer (that`s unless you enjoy reorganizing your sock drawer!) or counting your penny jar, basically whatever you find really boring.

The reason for this is also basic Behaviorism. You must not reward bad behavior. You must punish it, just like you must reward good behavior. In this case, you will be punishing your subconscious for not sleeping by giving it something boring. This will train your mind that staying awake equals boredom. So your mind will want to sleep when in bed. The boring activity will also help you `switch off`.

## 7) **Do not drink caffeine or alcohol after 3 pm.**

Try to avoid alcohol altogether, and don`t use it as a sleep aid. Caffeine will obviously keep you awake. If you drink lots of caffeine, try to cut down to five cups a day or less and don`t drink any after 3:00 PM. I don`t recommend cutting out caffeine altogether as tea, in particular, has various health benefits, including aiding cardiovascular functions which will improve general health and will therefore likely improve sleep. Just don't go overboard with caffeine.

Most people think alcohol helps us sleep better, but although alcohol makes us drowsy and sleepy, it makes it harder for most people to get a refreshing, deep sleep, which is the most important part of a good night's sleep.

Ever notice how after a boozy night, you can sleep longer than usual but feel more tired? I certainly do, so I try to limit the amount of alcohol I drink. If you`re a big drinker of alcohol and struggle with sleep, I suggest you cut down as much as possible. You will notice the benefits.

## 8) **Wear socks in bed... really.**

Recently researchers from The Netherlands have discovered that wearing socks in bed will help you get a much more restful sleep. They found that wearing socks increases the temperature of your feet which signal neurons in the brain to fall asleep. This is probably due to having warmer feet makes us feel more comfortable and secure. It certainly does work for me anyway.

You do want to make sure you are not too hot in bed, so although wearing socks is a good idea, try not to wear other items of clothing. I never sleep in a shirt, as I get too hot and restless and therefore wake up frequently. If you`re brave enough, I suggest wearing nothing but socks to go to sleep in. Just remember to put some clothes on when you get up in the morning if you have company. We don`t want you looking like a streakier!

9) **Laugh yourself to sleep**.

Stress is a major cause of depression, and depression is well-known by many to cause major sleep problems in some sufferers. In fact, I saw a GP on BBC news the other morning saying whenever a patient comes to him with sleep problems depression is often his first thought as to the cause.

This shows the importance of having a healthy mind. So, whenever you are stressed take a step back, ask yourself what you are stressed about, try to solve the problem before you get into bed, and laugh about it if possible.

Laughter is well-known as one of the most powerful antidotes to stress. Yes, admittedly, when you`re stressed it`s often hard to see the funny side, but you must try. Put on your favorite comedy, tell a joke, or just laugh for the sake of it. Even laughter that is false, is shown to lower blood pressure in some studies. Just the act of laughing is very powerful.

10) **Only go to bed when you are actually sleepy**.

Do not try to force sleep if you`re not actually sleepy. You`ll only increase your frustration and stress at not being able to sleep. What does stress cause - depression which causes a lack of sleep? A vicious circle. You may already be getting little sleep so don`t try and force it, believe me, it doesn't work. Wait till you are sleepy, then hit the hay.

All of these tips are derived from psychology, physiology, scientific research and my own experiences. This is just a simple guide of the best tips I've read and discovered and, most importantly tried and tested myself.

Try to incorporate one of these tips daily, and you will start to sleep better. I hope this article is useful to you all and you start getting a better nights' sleep.

# The Importance of Healthy Sleep

Healthy sleep is as important as diet, exercise and stress management for health. Many American's fail to make the effort to get healthy sleep, believing that sleep is expendable. Research is beginning to show us that this is not true. We are losing sleep at our own risk.

"There is plenty of compelling evidence supporting the argument that sleep is the most important predictor of how long you will live, perhaps more important than whether you smoke, exercise, or have high blood pressure or cholesterol levels."(1)

Believe it or not, getting healthy sleep...

* Can increase your ability to think clearly and function at your highest level

* Can boost athletic performance by 30%

* Improves your skin and appearance

* Helps you lose weight

* Improves your memory and ability to learn

* Decreases your risk of diabetes

* Helps to protect your heart and decrease your risk of heart disease

* Improves your ability to fight off infections

* Decreases your risk of accidents (2-4)

**The Benefits of Sleep:**

"We are not healthy unless our sleep is healthy." writes sleep research pioneer, William Dement, MD(1).

Intuitively, we've always known that sleep is important. "There's nothing better than a good night's sleep" is a common expression of this understanding. But for some reason, we don't listen to our own wisdom. As children, most of us had bedtimes that were the law of the household. Our parent's made sure that we got enough sleep. They knew what was good for us. As we got older most of us seem to have forgotten or ignored the value of sleep. We live in a culture that values industriousness, work, and productivity, and that frowns on lethargy.

Within just the past year (2008) there has been a surge of media attention on healthy sleep and insomnia. This is largely a result of more research coming out on the ill effects of insomnia for previously unsuspected conditions like heart disease, diabetes, cancer, obesity and weight gain. Researchers now suggest that insomnia is a major risk factor for these diseases.

Why are we losing so much healthy sleep?

**A major cause of lost sleep is stress and overwork.**

In stressful times in our life, a common reaction is to rev ourselves up to meet the demands placed upon us. Stresses may come and go in our individual lives. But now our entire society seems to be stressed. Almost no one would argue that we are now experiencing stress of historic proportions(circa 2008).

One of the first casualties of stress is healthy sleep. We Americans are struggling with insomnia more than ever. In 2005 a poll by the National Sleep Foundation reported that less than half of all Americans feel they get healthy sleep either every night or every other night(5).

Our nation's lack of healthy sleep is reflected by our use of sleep medications. Forty-nine million prescriptions for sleep medications were written in 2006(3). This was a 53% increase over the previous five years. The leading sleep drug is Ambien which accounted for 60% of sleep prescriptions in 2006, or $2,800,000,000 (2.8 billion) in sales. In 2006 drug companies spent $600,000,000 on advertising. The primary focus of all the advertising has been "destigmatizing sleeping pill use"(5).

While the major reason for all our sleeplessness is stress, our modern environment also discourages sleep.

Artificial light and man-made technologies give us many reasons to stay awake at night. Remember that for most of mankind's history the darkness of night put a real damper on staying awake to the wee hours. Our grandparents slept 1 1/2 hours more than we do each night according to Dr. Christopher Gillin, a psychiatrist, and a professor at the University of San Diego(6). He reports that one in three Americans complain of a bout of insomnia within the last year, and one in six consider their insomnia serious.

Thomas Edison himself, the inventor of the electric light bulb, believed that too much sleep was a bad thing. "The person who sleeps eight or ten hours a night is never fully asleep and never fully awake-he has only different degrees of doze through the 24 hours", said Edison. He felt that people got twice as much sleep as needed. Excess sleep caused them to be "unhealthy and inefficient"(1).

While Edison is known to have frequently slept only four hours a night, it is also reported that he also took frequent daytime naps. His total sleep time seems to have been close to 8 hours each 24 hours. Given Edison's personal philosophy it follows that he invented the electric light bulb. No single invention has so disrupted the human sleep cycle as electric lights.

The rhythm of healthy sleep and our biological clock

Our biological clock keeps time for our body's natural rhythm of sleep and awakening. It sets the timing of healthy sleep. Our body's clock can be upset by artificial light. Our body follows the day-night cycle by registering light through the eyes. This daily rhythm is called the circadian rhythm.

Every 24 hours as our earth rotates on its axis we experience this rhythm. It is the 24-hour repeating cycle that our lives are patterned after. The darkness of night stimulates our brain to release melatonin, the body's sleep hormone. Melatonin helps to induce sleep. Artificial lighting lowers melatonin secretion and can interfere with our ability to get to sleep.

The downside of our 24/7 Society

When our ancestors "burned the midnight oil" the light's intensity was not enough to disrupt our body's circadian rhythm. Light intensity is measured in lux. One lux is the amount of light given off by one candle. Researchers have shown that just 180 lux can reset or disrupt our biological clock. A 100-watt bulb at 10 feet distance emits 190 lux, which is enough to reset your biological clock.

With darkness, our eyes register less light. This signals our brain to release melatonin, the body's sleep hormone. Melatonin levels rise higher at night and drop in the daytime, all in response to the light coming into our eyes. This is how mankind experienced the day-night cycle for 1000's of years.

A glaring bright light at midnight tells your body that the sun is shining and as a result, your brain lowers melatonin levels. This disruption of melatonin can impact our sleep health. Melatonin has been shown to have many health benefits of its own. Lowering its levels in the body may also impact our health separate from the sleep issue. In our modern society, we are exposed to lots of stress and 24/7 activity. The combination of the two is seriously affecting our sleep. For most of us, our sleep is no longer healthy.

**What is a healthy sleep?**

Healthy sleep means you're getting enough sleep and that you are experiencing all of the stages of sleep in their proper amounts. How much sleep is enough? The consensus among sleep researchers is that adults need about eight hours a night.

Sleep researcher, Dr. William Dement puts it this way- "Generally people need to sleep one hour for every two hours awake, which means that most need around eight hours sleep a night. Of course, some people need more and some need less, and a few people seem to need a great deal more or less."(1) Before you begin to justify your chronic lapse of sleep, consider this powerful statement by Dr. Dement:

"Although sleep needs vary, people who sleep about eight hours, on average, tend to live longer".(1)

Other than the number of hours you get, how can you tell if you're getting enough sleep? The best way is to see how quickly you can fall asleep during the day if you're given a chance. This is how researchers measure sleep deprivation. The Multiple Sleep Latency Test is used by scientists to assess the level of an individual's sleep deprivation.

Research subjects are given a place to lie down comfortably in a quiet, dark room in the middle of the day. The volunteer's brain waves are monitored to see if and when they go to sleep. The test lasts just 20 minutes. Research subjects are given a place to lie down comfortably in a quiet, dark room in the middle of the day. The volunteer's brain waves are monitored to see if and when they go to sleep. The test lasts just 20 minutes.

If the subject falls asleep in under 5 minutes this represents a severe sleep deficiency. These subject's "physical and mental reactions are often very impaired"(1). Falling asleep in between 5 and 10 minutes is considered being "borderline" sleep deprived. Falling asleep between 10 and 15 minutes indicates an acceptable amount of sleep need. Falling asleep in 15 to 20 minutes or not at all suggests that the subject has an excellent level of alertness.

Another way to see how sleep deprived you are is to look at how sleepy you are. The sleepier you are the more you need sleep, right? This evaluation, called the Epworth sleepiness scale (8) is accurate whether you're someone who needs more or less than eight hours. If you're sleepy, you're just not getting enough sleep.

The normal sleep cycle.

The other part of getting healthy sleep is having a normal sleep cycle. This means that you go through all of the cycles of sleep and experience each of them for a sufficient amount of time.

There are four stages of sleep and REM. Stages 1 through 4 are a progression from falling asleep (stage 1), into the light sleep (stage 2) and then deep sleep (stages 3 and 4). During deep sleep, the body is in a profoundly relaxed state. Muscle tension is relaxed, blood pressure slows, and heart rate and breathing are diminished. During deep sleep, the body secretes pulses of human growth hormone.

Human growth hormone is sometimes called the hormonal fountain of youth because of its rejuvenating qualities. Each night your body repairs and restores itself under the direction of human growth hormone. After going into deep sleep one emerges into REM sleep. During REM sleep there is Rapid Eye Movement. REM is when we dream. Researchers have found that REM sleep seems to help us remember what we learned the day before.

# References


(1) Dement, William C., Vaughan, Christopher. The Promise of Sleep. Introduction. © 1999, Dell Publishing, NY, NY. William Dement, M.D. is a pioneer in sleep research who has worked to promote awareness of the epidemic of sleeplessness and its ill effects.

(2) Susan Brink (2000, October). Sleepless Society In staying up half the night, we may risk our health. U.S. News & World Report, 129(15), 62-72.

(3) Well-Rested Olympians Ready to Go for Gold. (2006, February). USA Today, 134(2729), 15.

(4) Lauren Wiener, Hollace Schmidt. (2007, March). your new #1 stay-healthy mission: get more sleep. Shape, 26(7), 98,100-102.

(5) Mooallem, Jon. The Sleep-Industrial Complex. New York Times, November 18, 2007.

(6) From published notes of a radio interview the week of March 31, 1999, Lichenstein Creative Media, The Infinite Mind.

(7) The Free Dictionary by Farlex.

(8) From Wikipedia, keyword: Epworth Sleepiness Scale